YOUR KNOWLEDGE HAS VALUE

AF140751

- We will publish your bachelor's and
  master's thesis, essays and papers

- Your own eBook and book -
  sold worldwide in all relevant shops

- Earn money with each sale

Upload your text at www.GRIN.com
and publish for free

G R I N ☺

Bibliographic information published by the German National Library:

The German National Library lists this publication in the National Bibliography; detailed bibliographic data are available on the Internet at http://dnb.dnb.de .

Imprint:

Copyright © 2016 GRIN Verlag, Open Publishing GmbH
Print and binding: Books on Demand GmbH, Norderstedt Germany
ISBN: 9783668222953

This book at GRIN:

http://www.grin.com/en/e-book/321604/does-cell-phone-use-increase-the-risk-of-brain-tumors

Amir Hossein Mortazavi Entesab, Naina Sawal

Does cell phone use increase the risk of brain tumors?

Review of 11 studies

GRIN Publishing

GRIN - Your knowledge has value

Since its foundation in 1998, GRIN has specialized in publishing academic texts by students, college teachers and other academics as e-book and printed book. The website www.grin.com is an ideal platform for presenting term papers, final papers, scientific essays, dissertations and specialist books.

Visit us on the internet:

http://www.grin.com/

http://www.facebook.com/grincom

http://www.twitter.com/grin_com

Mobile phone usage and the risk of brain tumors

Naina Sawal B.Sc.,

Amir Hossein Mortazavi Entesab M.D., M.Sc.

CONTENTS

ABSTRACT

Purpose: This literature review investigated the possible association between the use of mobile phones and brain tumors.

Methods: In brief, 11 publications were retrieved from JSTOR, PubMed, Google Scholar, and Summon in order to compare the association between the usage of mobile phones in patients with a brain tumor and those without. Papers published in English, and after 2001 were selected for. There was no limit on age, gender, geographical location and type of brain tumor.

Results: For regular mobile phone usage, the combined odds ratios (OR) (95% confidence intervals) for three studies was: 1.5 (1.2-1.8); 1.3 (0.95-1.9); and 1.1 (0.8-1.4), respectively. Furthermore, the odds ratio did not increase, regardless of mobile phone use duration. Additionally, Lonn et al (2005) observed that the risk also did not significantly increase when assessing the laterality (ipsilateral or contralateral) of the tumor in relation to side of head used for the mobile phone. Kan et al (2008) observed an OR of 1.22 when comparing analog phone to digital phone use.

Conclusion: This review concluded that there is no current association between mobile phone use and the development of brain tumors. Although certain studies speak in favor of an increased risk, many are plagued with either: sampling bias, misclassification bias, or issues concerning risk estimates. Further research needs to be done in order to evaluate the long-term effect of mobile phone usage on the risk of developing a brain tumor.

INTRODUCTION

In the past 20 years, the use of cellular telephones has increased exponentially in today's society, with greater than 5.3 billion mobile subscriptions worldwide (Cardis, 2011). Consequently, numerous concerns have been raised regarding the connection between radiofrequency signals emitted from these devices and the possible risk of developing chronic diseases. Although current guidelines state that mobile phones emit energy levels far too low to cause any deleterious health effects, there has been growing debate as to whether a relative risk has not been established due to the different levels of exposure when the research was initially conducted. Especially since early mobile phones were developed with an analog technology, and emitted radiofrequency waves of only 800-900 megahertz (Mhz) (Linet, 2013) and recent years have seen it become replaced with a digital technology which utilizes much higher radiofrequencies (ranging up to 2200 Mhz) (Linet, 2013)

As such, numerous attempts have been made to evaluate this connection based on the standard of mobile phone usage today – with much of the research focusing on the effects of mobile phone usage and the development of tumors, particularly in the head and neck region. In particular, research has focused on tumors particular to the temporal area of the brain – a region proposed to experience the most exposure to mobile phone radiation – including tumors like, meningiomas, gliomas, and acoustic neuromas (Christensen, 2003). The current argument in favor of an association proposes that although low frequency radiation is non-ionizing - in that it does not damage DNA - if presented at high enough levels the radiofrequency radiation can induce a thermal change in tissues and thereby stimulate tumor growth (Linet, 2013).

Yet despite this growing database of scientific research, the topic still remains controversial. While some case-control studies have purported to find a connection between brain tumors and increased mobile phone usage via a tumor "promoter" effect (Hardell, 2003), other case-control studies find no short-term effects of cell phone electromagnetic field exposure on brain pathology (Mandala, 2014). At present, any evidence arguing for a causal relationship between mobile phone use and the development of brain tumors has been found to be inconclusive upon further critical examination (Kundi 2009).

3

In this study, we compared the observed patterns for brain tumor incidence trends in a variety of publications, particularly those of a meta-analysis or case control nature, in order to investigate the association between mobile phone use and the risk of brain tumor development.

METHODS

Incidence data was gathered from a variety of databases including: JSTOR, Pub med database (http://www.ncbi.nlm.nih.gov/pubmed), Google Scholar (http://www.scholar.google.com) and Summon. The keywords specified to search for the articles include: Cellular phone, Cancer, Tumor, Brain, Mobile phone, Short term, Long term, Cross-sectional, Meta-analysis, Radiofrequencies, Glioma, Meningioma, and Schwannoma. In order to ensure the information presented is valid and applicable to the topic, all of the articles chosen will be published between 2001 and 2014. Additionally, due to the lack of consensus on research areas on this topic, the study populations selected will include both male and female cellular phone users of any age group, in any geographic setting. Lastly, in order to avoid any misunderstandings in discourse, only papers published in English will be selected for. Non-human studies were discarded.

To assess for a possible causal relationship between mobile phone use and cancer, all of the data gathered from the publications and analyzed in order to construct an evidence table based on the findings of each study. Those studies demonstrating the relationship between mobile phone use and brain tumor development were assessed by their subgroups in order to gather information based on tumor histology, tumor location (ipsilateral or contralateral), type of phone (analog or digital), and amount of use. If there are no valid counter arguments against a particular piece of evidence for an association then causation is suggested. However, when the evidence is insufficient the confidence in a causal relationship decreases.

RESULTS

In brief, 14 articles were selected for this review paper. Five of those articles were a level 4, six articles were level 3, and two were level 1. One of the level 3 studies focused on brain cancer incidence trends in the United States, specifically in its Caucasian population (2010). Similarly, Benson et al (2013) examined the incidence of intracranial tumors in middle-aged women in the United Kingdom. Additionally, while Cardis et al (2011) conducted a case-control study solely on patients with newly diagnosed acoustic neuromas in 13 countries using a common protocol; Schuz et al (2011) used two Danish nationwide cohort studies to assess acoustic neuroma occurrence. Another the level 4 articles was centered on cell phone use and the implications to brain tumor risk in adolescents with a mean age of 12.3 years (Aydin, 2011). The remaining publications selected assessed the risk of any intracranial tumor with increased mobile phone usage, regardless of gender, age, or race. As such, the chosen articles were also targeted to allow for direct comparisons, with respect of mobile phone usage, and its subsequent radiation exposure, to the development of brain tumors in individuals in the control group who were found to be without a brain tumor.

Study Design	Number of Studies
Meta Analysis	5
Case Control	6
Review	2
Log Linear Model	1

Table 1: Summary of study designs reviewed

The articles analyzed focused on a variety of factors for their assessment of causality. Two articles measured the duration of cell phone usage and cancer incidence rate. Five out of eleven articles addressed tumor location (ipsilateral or contralateral) compared to patient mobile phone. Four out of eleven articles evaluated the risk of developing more than one type brain tumor with mobile phone use. Three out of eleven articles compared the cancer incidence risk between analogy and digital phones. Further detail on the articles can be found in the evidence table (See Appendix A, Table A.1).

Lahkola et al (2006) examined the effect of mobile phone use on a risk of developing a variety of intracranial tumors by conducting a meta-analysis involving 12 studies (Figure 1). The odds ratio (OR) was found to be insignificant at 0.98 (95% confidence interval; CI = 0.83-1.16) for all intracranial tumors related to

5

mobile phone use. For gliomas, the pooled OR was 0.96 (95% CI 0.78-1.18), for meningiomas it was 0.87 (95% CI 0.72-1.05), and for acoustic neuromas it was 1.07 (95% CI 0.89-1.30). Kan et al (2008) conducted a similar study examining the OR for high-grade gliomas, meningiomas, and acoustic neuromas. The pooled OR was valued at being lower than 1, and the odds ratio for low-grade glioma was found to be insignificant with a OR = 1.14 (95% confidence interval; CI = 0.91 to 1.43] (Kan, 2008).

Similarly, Johansen et al (2001) analyzed various intracranial and body tumors and their association with mobile phone use (Figure 1). The standard incidence ratio (SIR) for brain tumors was 0.86 (95% confidence interval; CI = 0.83 to 0.90) in males, therefore showing no evidence of an increased risk for tumors of the brain.

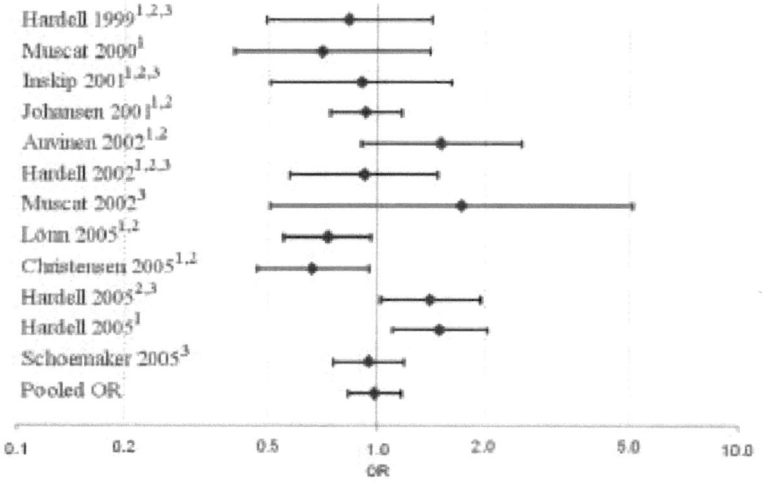

Figure 1: Pooled odds ratio of original studies and meta-analysis of mobile phone use and intracranial tumors. Studies including gliomas (1), meningiomas (2), acoustic neuromas (3).

6

When measuring brain tumor incidence risk based on location relative to cell phone placement, Larjavaara et al (2010) found that on a case analysis basis, tumors were found to be located contralateral to cell phone placement, but not in a manner that was statistically significant. The odds ratio for this brain tumor risk among contralateral regular phone users (at least 1 call per week for a period of 6 months or more) was higher than the OR of ipsilateral regular phone users OR = 0.87 and OR = 0.82, (95% CI), respectively. Additionally, it was concluded that although nearly 97% to 99% of the energy from a mobile phone is absorbed by the hemisphere within 5 cm of the handset, there was no excess of gliomas found in the temporal lobe among regular users compared to the never regular users (28% vs. 33% of the locations in the cerebral lobes) (Larjavaara 2010).

Christensen et al (2003) also did not detect an increase in frequency on a particular side of the head relative mobile phone placement, nor did they find that tumor size correlated with the pattern of cell phone usage (Table 2).

Handedness and laterality of cellular telephone use	Cases		Controls	
	No.	%	No.	%
Same side	19	42	57	59
Opposite side	14	31	30	31
Ambidextrous*	3	7	4	4
No preferred side	9	20	6	6

Table 2: Handedness and acoustic neuroma incidence among cancer patients and controls in Denmark, 2000-2002 (Christensen, 2003)

Contradictory to this claim is the international INTERPHONE case-control study which followed the tumor development in a specific cohort of users with a cumulative mobile phone usage of greater than 1640 hours (Cardis, 2011), and found an OR=2.33 (CI: 1.23-4.40) and an OR=0.72 (CI: 0.34-1.53) relative to ipsilateral vs. contralateral use, respectively (Cardis, 2011). But it is important to note that this causality only held up in the high exposure cohort, as the cohorts with a lower levels of exposure all exhibited an OR less than 1, regardless of laterality (Cardis, 2011). Similarly, Schoemaker et al (2005) also found an OR-0.9 (95%

confidence interval: CI=0.7-1.1) for the development of acoustic neuromas within the first 10 years of mobile phone usage. Both Schuz et al (2011) and Christensen et al (2005) found there to be no increased risk in the development of brain tumors with mobile phone usage of greater than 10 years.

Another factor addressed was the affect of the analog vs. digital cell phones on the incidence of brain tumors. Johansen et al (2001) found that the SIRs for tumors of the brain and nervous system were not related to duration of usage, or cellular telephone system used, whether digital or analog (Table 3). Lahkola et al (2006) conducted a meta-analysis to pool estimates for the use of analog and digital telephones, finding that both were slightly above one, with analog telephones having a pooled OR slightly greater than that of digital telephones; Therefore proving to be insignificant. Schoemaker et al (2005) also came to the same conclusion in their analysis that there was no causality of an increased risk of developing acoustic neuromas amongst analog or digital cell phone users.

Lahkola et al (2006) also conducted a regression analysis of the pooled data, and found that there was no increased risk of intracranial tumors with duration of mobile usage (regression coefficient 0.0072, P=0.41), (Figure 2). Aydin et al (2012) compared the incidence of brain and nervous system tumors in children ages 5-19 living in Nordic countries relative to the proportion of regular mobile phone users (Figure 3), concluding there to be no variance from past trends. Benson et al (2013) also conducted a large prospective study measuring mobile phone usage amongst middle-aged women in the UK, and found that there was no increased risk with a relative risk (RR) of 1.01 (95% CI = 0.9-1.14). Similarly, Christensen et al (2005) reported that non-mobile phone users actually had an increased mean tumor size in each of the three types of brain tumors measured (meningioma, low-grade glioma, high-grade glioma), relative to regular mobile phone users.

Exposure variable	Brain and nervous tumors				Leukemia			
	Obs	Exp	SIR	95% CI	Obs	Exp	SIR	95% CI
Total	154	161.3	1.0	0.8 to 1.1	84	86.2	1.0	0.8 to 1.2
Latency,† y								
<1	43	55.2	0.8	0.6 to 1.1	29	28.4	1.0	0.7 to 1.5
1–4	87	83.1	1.1	0.9 to 1.3	44	44.1	1.0	0.7 to 1.3
≥5	24	23.0	1.0	0.7 to 1.6	11	13.7	0.8	0.4 to 1.4
Trend test‡				$P = .16$				$P = .55$
Age at entry, y								
0–49	97	96.2	1.0	0.8 to 1.2	36	34.7	1.0	0.7 to 1.4
50–64	41	52.7	0.8	0.6 to 1.1	31	36.6	0.9	0.6 to 1.2
≥65	16	12.4	1.3	0.7 to 1.3	17	14.9	1.2	0.7 to 1.8
Trend test‡				$P = .90$				$P = .96$
Cellular telephone system used								
Analogue	84	81.0	1.0	0.8 to 1.3	39	46.1	0.9	0.6 to 1.6
Analogue and digital	20	15.0	1.3	0.8 to 2.1	10	7.2	1.4	0.7 to 2.5
Digital	50	56.1	0.9	0.7 to 1.2	35	28.1	1.2	0.9 to 1.7
Duration of digital subscription,§ y								
<1	12	17.5	0.7	0.4 to 1.2	10	8.3	1.2	0.6 to 2.2
1–2	29	31.1	0.9	0.6 to 1.3	19	15.8	1.2	0.7 to 1.9
≥3	9	7.5	1.2	0.6 to 2.3	6	4.1	1.5	0.5 to 3.2
Trend test‡				$P = .19$				$P = .75$

Table 3: Analog phone and Digital phone use and risk of brain and nervous system tumors.

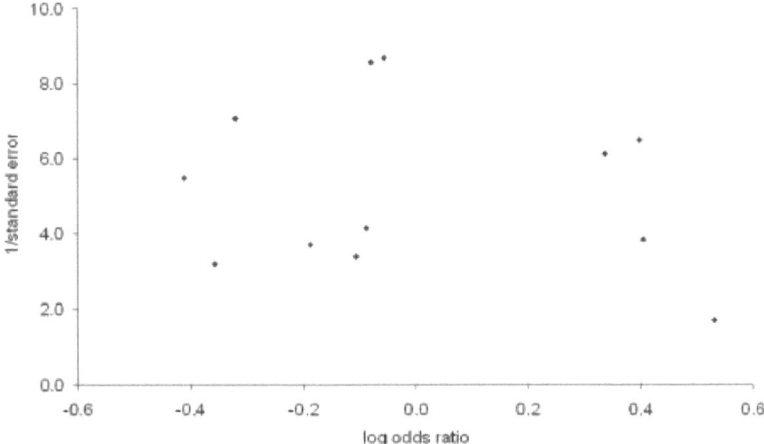

Figure 2: Funnel plot of studies included in the meta-analysis, showing no evidence of publication bias concerning intracranial tumors and mobile phone use.

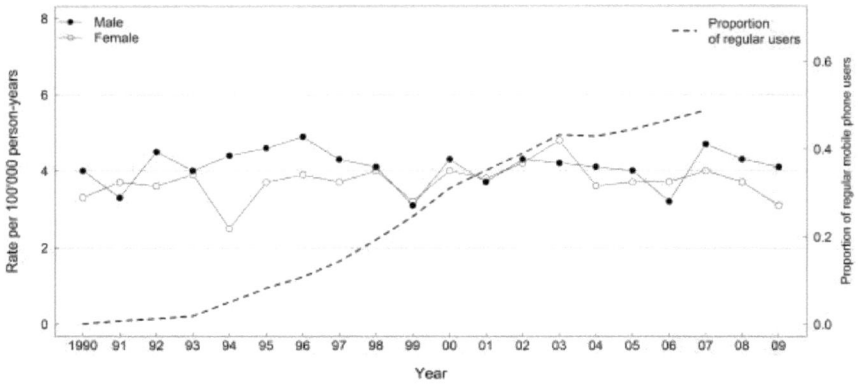

<u>Figure 3</u>: Age-standardized (age 5-19) incidence rates for brain and central nervous system tumors in children living in Nordic Countries.

DISCUSSION

This paper pooled the published risk estimates of 11 publications in order to assess their conclusions regarding the risk of developing brain tumors relative to the usage of mobile phones. By measuring several subgroup factors like tumor size and variety, brain tumor laterality, mobile phone use duration, and mobile phone type it was concluded that there is no increased risk in the development of brain tumors relative to the use of mobile phones. These findings are in line with previously conducted meta-analysis studies on the subject.

Both Cardis et al (2011) and Schuz et al (2013) conducted cohort studies, which concluded that there was no increased risk in developing acoustic neuromas in long-term mobile phone users compared to both short term and nonsubscribers. Schuz et al (2013) also found that the groups did not differ in regard to tumor incidence rates, tumor size, and laterality of tumor location with respect to cell phone usage. According to Benson et al (2013), there was found to be no association with an increased risk of glioma, meningioma, total cancer or cancer at 18 other specific sites in middle-aged UK women. Although certain authors like Benson et al (2013) also propose that there is may be an increased risk with longer mobile phone usage, there is no such pathologic causality evident in respect to other research on the same subject thereby suggesting a possible information bias (Christensen, 2005).

Additionally, the statistically significant disparity amongst the results from these different studies in the main analysis of the various brain tumors studied suggest that this variation could be due to procedural or measurement bias. It is likely that the increased risk causality found in the INTERPHONE study may be due to the recall bias found with self-reporting (Benson, 2013). Schoemaker et al (2005) noted that recall bias may result in cases over-reporting ipsilateral mobile use because of the belief that it caused the development of the tumor. This would not only increase the risk for ipsilateral use, but also decrease the risk for contralateral use (Schoemaker, 2005). Cardis et al (2011) attempted to rule out this bias by ensuring that cases were not aware of the exact tumor location prior to discussion about cell phone use, but it was also noted that mobile users with the least exposure tended to underestimate their usage. Similarly, Aydin et al (2011) compared operator recorded data to self-reported mobile phone use, and found the former subset of participants to have a higher reliability thus allowing for the reduction recall bias. Cardis et al (2011)

Johansen et al (2001) suggests a possible confounding effect based on occupation or socioeconomic status, as police officers may have a greater risk due to their exposure to radar guns. Kundi et al (2008) also noted that mobile phone use is not randomly distributed within a population, as usage patterns vary depending on sex, age, occupation, and socioeconomic status. Schoemaker et al (2005) attempted to match participants by age and usage in order to bypass any selection bias They noted that since childhood brain tumors have a relatively low occurrence rate, the high exposure to mobile phones in adolescents did not produce any deviation from the expected values (Schoemaker, 2005). Christensen et al (2004) also matched their respective cohorts based on socioeconomic data gathered from registries in order to minimize selection bias.

Additionally, much of smaller scale research arguing in favor of causality has problems in addition to selection bias (Christensen, 2005), as is seen with Benson et al (2013) and their inconsistent measurement amongst users. This sampling bias results in large confidence intervals, which make establishing causality incredibly difficult (Aydin, 2011). Kundi et al (2008) notes that very few studies have conducted long-term studies with users mirroring the same pattern of usage. Although Johansen et al (2001) conducted a nationwide study following mobile phone usage over the course of 13 years; the authors note that the exposure levels between 1982-1995 vary greatly from the time of publication. However, Inskip et al (2010) followed mobile phone patterns and incidence trends well into the 21st century amongst what is arguably the cohort with the highest exposure and found there to be no difference among trends. If anything the incident rates have been decreasing, which may be attributable to earlier diagnosis with advanced medical techniques (Inskip, 2010).

Benson et al (2013) proposes that this limitation may lead to underestimation of a relative risk towards the null since those diagnosed with a tumor may have experienced tumor related symptoms (headache, hearing loss) prior to diagnosis - which caused them to either change their amount of usage or change the side upon which they hold their phone. Similarly these symptoms could also result in early detection thereby increasing the risk for short-term users (Schoemaker, 2005). Cardis et al (2011) found that upon adjusting mobile phone use 1 year prior to the reference date, they allowed for a similar latent period between first exposure and tumor diagnosis. This allowed them to adjust for any behavioral changes due to prodromal symptoms, as there was no change observed between tumor laterality and expected incidence rates. Consequently, Aydin et al (2011) noted that the OR for brain tumors in cases restricted to tumors of the temporal and frontal lobes were not increased despite their variance in exposure levels, thereby suggesting that no relationship exists.

Lahkola et al (2006) was cites inconsistent exposure classifications as making it difficult for pooling studies to be conducted in a comparable fashion. While some studies compare analog and digital phones in different subsets, others do not make this differentiation (Lakhola, 2006). Kundi et al (2008) affirms that such variety in measurement makes it difficult to evaluate whether or not increased exposure has an effect on tumor laterality. Kan et al (2008) noted a possible confounding relationship between the type of mobile phone and usage latency. Lakhola et al (2008) also reported similarities in Sweden amongst the OR of long-term user risk (greater than 5 years) and the OR of analog phones, 0.83 and 0.9

respectively (Lakhola 2008). However since the switch to digital phones has been fairly recent, this may be a conclusion subject to change in the long-term.

In summary, the results of this review are applicable to any population as data from each publication came from a variety of populations. Consequently, at present there exists no evidence of a causal relationship between mobile phone use and brain tumors throughout a variety of cohorts. Although there is some weak evidence in favor of a causal relationship in some in vitro studies, overall in vitro data as proven inconclusive. However, it is important to note that this does not rule out any causal relationship in the long-term since it can take many years for carcinogens to produce a change in pathology. More research on this topic should focus on the long-term applications amongst large population studies in order to give more confidence as to the overall relationship.

CONCLUSION

Upon review of current literature, there was not found to be any evidence of a causal relationship between mobile phone usage and the development of brain tumors. Despite the large-scale studies of Hardell and colleagues, the lack of investigation on the long-term effects of cell phone usage makes it difficult to asses whether any evidence proposing a causal relationship is based on a definite linkage or merely a chance occurrence. Future studies focusing on long-term mobile phone exposure (10 years or more) need to be conducted in order to shed light on this controversial matter, and hopefully tip the scale in a definitive direction.

Table 4: Evidence table (Strategy for synthesizing the data)

First Author	Date of Publication	Study Design	Level of Evidence	Study Population	Therapy or Exposure	Outcome/ Results
Martha Linet	December 2013	Review	1	Cellular phone users	Analogue and digital cellular phones	Data is inconclusive to suggest a linkage between factors.
Peter Kan	June 7, 2007	Meta Analysis	3	Cellular phone users	Analogue or digital cellular phones	No overall increased risk of brain tumors among cellular phone users
Michael Kundi	September 26, 2008	Review	1	Cellular phone users	Cellular phone	The overall evidence speaks in favor of an increased risk, but its magnitude cannot be assessed at present because of insufficient information on long-term use.
Peter D. Inskip	July 16, 2010	Log linear model	3	Caucasian patients diagnosed with brain tumor	Radiofrequency radiation from cellular phones	Incident data does not provide support to the view that cellular phone use causes brain cancer
Suvi Larjavaara	February 12, 2011	Case-Case analysis	4	Glioma Brain tumor patients and a control group	Cellular phones	There is no association between glioma development and regular mobile phone use regardless of duration of use and laterality.
J Schuz	August 15, 2011	Meta-analysis	4	Cellular phone users	Cellular phones	Currently there's no correlation between cell phone use and vestibular schwannomas
Denis Aydin	April 2, 2012	Case-control study	3	Children and adolescents aged 7-19 years diagnosed with brain tumor	Mobile phones	Absence of exposure – response relationship

First Author	Date of Publication	Study Design	Level of Evidence	Study Population	Therapy or Exposure	Outcome/ Results
H. Collatz Christensen	April, 2005	Case-control study	4	Patients with Glioma or meningioma aged 20 to 69	Cellular phones	No association between use of cellular telephones and risk for glioma or meningioma
Elisabeth Cardis	August 23, 2011	Case-control Study	3	Patients with newly diagnosed acoustic neuroma	Mobile telephone	No increase in the risk of acoustic neuroma with the use of mobile phones regularly
M. Mandala	2014	Case-control study	3	Cellular phone users	Mobile and portable telephones	Mobile phone use is not related to risk of auditory nerve damage or tumor development.
Anna Lahkola	2006	Meta-analysis	4	Long term mobile phone users (more than 5 years)	Mobile phones	No substantial increase in risk of intracranial tumors from mobile phone use for a period of at least 5 years
M. Schoemaker	August 30, 2005	Meta-analysis	3	Patients diagnosed with acoustic neuroma	Mobile phones	No risk of acoustic neuroma in the first 10 years after starting mobile phone use
Victoria Benson	March 28, 2013	Case-control study	1	Female patients diagnosed with intracranial tumors	Cellular phones	Mobile phone use was not associated with increased incidence of glioma, meningioma, or non-CNS cancers.
S Lonn	March 15, 2005	Meta-analysis	4	Cellular phone users with brain tumors	Cellular phones	Mobile phone use is unrelated to an increased risk of glioma or meningioma use.

LITERATURE CITED

1. S. Lonn, A Ahlbom, P Hall, M Feychting (2005). Long term mobile phone use and brain tumor risk. Am J Epidemiology, Volume 161, Issue 6, 526-535.

2. Peter Kan, Sara E. Simonsen, Joseph L. Lyon, John R. W. Kestle. (June 7, 2007). Cellular phone use and brain tumor: a meta-analysis. Journal of Neuro-oncology, Volume 86, Number 1, 71-78.

3. Martha Linet, Peter, Inskip. (2010). Cellular telephone use and cancer risk. Rev Environ Health, Volume 25, Issue 1, 51-55.

4. Michael Kundi. (September 2008). The controversy about a possible relationship between mobile phone use and cancer: Environmental Health Perspective 2009, Volume 117, Issue 10, pages 316-324.

5. Peter D. Inskip, Robert N. Hoover, and Susan S. Devesa. (June 7, 2010). Brain cancer incidence trends in relation to cellular telephone use in the United States. Neuro Oncology 2010, Volume 12, Issue 11, 1147-1151.

6. Suvi Larjavaara, Joachim Schuz, Anthony Swerdlow, Maria Feychting, Christoffer Johansen. (February 2, 2011). Location of gliomas in relation to mobile telephone use: a case-case and case specular analysis. Journal of Epidemiology, Volume 174, Issue 1, 2-11.

7. J. Schuz, M. Steding-Jessen, S Hansen, SE Stangerup, P Caye-Thomasen. (August 2011). Long-term mobile phone use and the risk of vestibular schwannoma: a Danish nationwide cohort study. American Journal of Epidemiology, Volume 174, Issue 4, 416-422.

8. Denis Aydin, Maria Feychting, Joachim Schüz, Tore Tynes, Tina Veje Andersen, Lisbeth Samsø Schmidt (April 2, 2012). Childhood brain tumors and use of mobile phones: comparison of a case-control study with incidence data. Environmental Health, Volume 11, Issue 35, 1-3.

9. H. Collatz Christensen, J. Schüz, M. Kosteljanetz, H. Skovgaard Poulsen, J.D. Boice, J.K. McLaughlin, C. Johansen. (April 2004). Cellular telephones and risk for acoustic neuroma. American Journal of Epidemiology, Volume 159, Issue 3, 277-283.

10. Elisabeth Cardis, BK Armstrong. (June 9, 2011). Risk of brain tumors in relation to estimated RF dose from mobile phones: results from five Interphone countries. Occup Environ Med, Volume 68, 631-640.

11. M. Mandala, V Colletti, L Sacchetto, P Manganotti, S Ramat, A Marcocci. (January 2014). Effect of Bluetooth headset and mobile phone electromagnetic fields on the human auditory nerve. Laryngoscope, Volume 124, Issue 1, 255-259.

12. Victoria Benson, Kirstin Pirie, Joachim Schuz, Gilliam Reeves, Valerie Beral, Jane Green. (2013). Mobile phone use and risk of brain neoplasms and other cancers: prospective study. International Journal of Epidemiology, Volume 42, Issue 3, 792-802.

13. Anna Lahkola, Karl Tokola, Anssi Auvinen. (2006). Meta-analysis of mobile phone use and intracranial tumors. Scand J Work Environ Health, Volume 32, no. 3, 171-177.

14. MJ Schoemaker, AJ Swerdlow, A Ahlbom, A Auvinen, KG Blaasaas, E Cardis. (August 30, 2005). Mobile phone use and risk of acoustic neuroma: results of the interphone case-control study in five North European countries, Volume 93, Issue 1, 842-848.

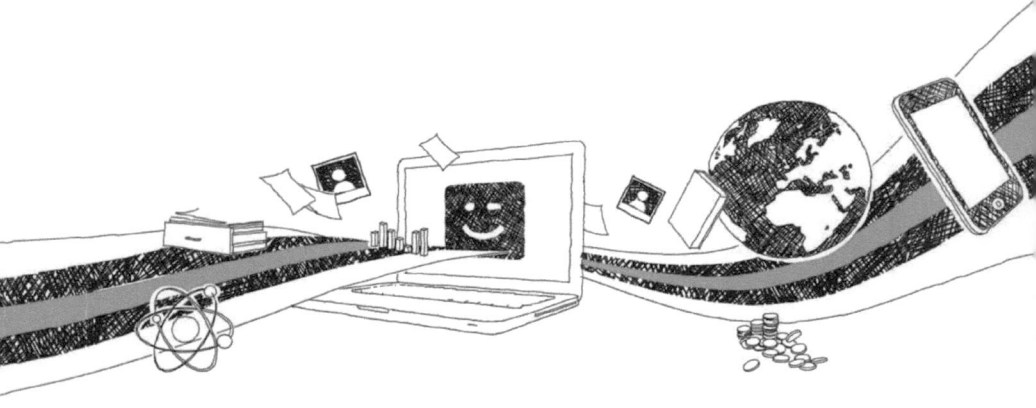
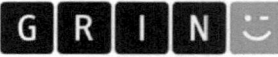